Bananas Everyday

A Cookbook for Beginners With Over 100 Exquisite Recipes That You Can Easily Make At Home

Paul Gidney

SPECIAL DISCLAIMER

All the information's included in this book are given for instructive, informational and entertainment purposes, the author can claim to share very good quality recipes but is not headed for the perfect data and uses of the mentioned recipes, in fact the information's are not intent to provide dietary advice without a medical consultancy.

The author does not hold any responsibility for errors, omissions or contrary interpretation of the content in this book.

It is recommended to consult a medical practitioner before to approach any kind of diet, especially if you have a particular health situation, the author isn't headed for the responsibility of these situations and everything is under the responsibility of the reader, the author strongly recommend to preserve the health taking all precautions to ensure ingredients are fully cooked.

All the trademarks and brands used in this book are only mentioned to clarify the sources of the information's and to describe better a topic and all the trademarks and brands mentioned own their copyrights and they are not related in any way to this document and to the author.

This document is written to clarify all the information's of publishing purposes and cover any possible issue.

This document is under copyright and it is not possible to reproduce any part of this content in every kind of digital or printable document. All rights reserved.

Table Of Contents

Table Of Contents

Table Of Contents

Banana Cream Pie I

Ingredients

3/4 cup white sugar 1/3
cup all-purpose flour 1/4
teaspoon salt
2 cups milk
3 egg yolks, beaten
2 tablespoons butter
1 1/4 teaspoons vanilla extract
1 (9 inch) pie crust, baked
4 bananas, sliced

Directions

In a saucepan, combine the sugar, flour, and salt. Add milk in gradually while stirring gently. Cook over medium heat, stirring constantly, until the mixture is bubbly. Keep stirring and cook for about 2 more minutes, and then remove from the burner.

Stir a small quantity of the hot mixture into the beaten egg yolks, and immediately add egg yolk mixture to the rest of the hot mixture. Cook for 2 more minutes; remember to keep stirring. Remove the mixture from the stove, and add butter and vanilla. Stir until the whole thing has a smooth consistency.

Slice bananas into the cooled baked pastry shell. Top with pudding mixture.

Bake at 350 degrees F (175 degrees C) for 12 to 15 minutes. Chill for an hour.

Mocha Chocolate Chip Banana Muffins

Ingredients

1 cup margarine
1 1/4 cups white sugar
1 egg
3 ripe bananas
1 tablespoon instant coffee granules, dissolved in
1 tablespoon water
1 teaspoon vanilla extract
2 1/4 cups all-purpose flour
1/4 teaspoon salt
1 teaspoon baking powder
1 teaspoon baking soda
1 cup semisweet chocolate chips

Directions

Preheat oven to 350 degrees F (175 degrees C).

Blend butter or margarine, sugar, egg, banana, dissolved coffee, and vanilla in food processor for 2 minutes. Add flour, salt, baking powder, and soda, and blend just until flour disappears. Add chocolate chips and mix in with wooden spoon. Spoon mixture into 15 to 18 paper-lined muffin cups.

Bake for 25 minutes. Cool on wire racks.

Whole Grain Healthy Banana Bread

Ingredients

3/4 cup SPLENDA® Sugar Blend
3/4 cup flax seed meal
5 ripe bananas, mashed
1/4 cup skim milk
1/4 cup low-fat sour cream
2 teaspoons egg whites
2 cups whole wheat flour
1 teaspoon baking soda
1/2 teaspoon salt

Directions

Preheat the oven to 350 degrees F (175 degrees C). Grease and a 9x5 inch loaf pan.

In a medium bowl, mix together the sugar blend, flax meal, bananas, milk, sour cream and egg whites until well blended. Combine the flour, baking soda and salt; stir into the banana mixture until moistened. Spoon into prepared loaf pan.

Bake for 1 hour and 10 minutes in the preheated oven, or until a toothpick inserted into the crown of the loaf comes out clean.

Chocolate-Banana Tofu Pudding

Ingredients

1 banana, broken into chunks
1 (12 ounce) package soft silken tofu
1/4 cup confectioners' sugar
5 tablespoons unsweetened cocoa powder
3 tablespoons soy milk
1 pinch ground cinnamon

Directions

Place the banana, tofu, sugar, cocoa powder, soy milk, and cinnamon into a blender. Cover, and puree until smooth. Pour into individual serving dishes, and refrigerate for 1 hour before serving.

Banana Split Cake V

Ingredients

2 cups all-purpose flour
1 3/4 cups margarine, softened
1/2 cup chopped pecans
2 eggs
2 cups confectioners' sugar
6 bananas
1 (20 ounce) can crushed pineapple, drained
2 pints fresh strawberries
1 (16 ounce) container frozen whipped topping, thawed

Directions

Preheat oven to 375 degrees F (190 degrees C).

In a large bowl, combine flour, 3/4 cup margarine and chopped pecans. Press into the bottom of a 9x13 inch pan. Bake in preheated oven for 20 mintes. Remove from oven and allow to cool.

In a large bowl, combine 1 cup margarine, eggs and confectioners' sugar. Beat with an electric mixer for 6 minutes or until fluffy.
Spread over cooled crust. Slice bananas and arrange on filling. Slice strawberries and layer over bananas. Cover with whipped topping and garnish with a sprinkling of chopped nuts.

Lower Fat Banana Nut Bread

Ingredients

3/4 cup fat free sour cream
4 egg whites
1/4 cup chopped walnuts
1/3 cup raisins (optional)
2 teaspoons baking powder
2 teaspoons baking soda
6 very ripe bananas, mashed
2 tablespoons reduced fat margarine
1 tablespoon vanilla extract
1 teaspoon salt
2/3 cup packed light brown sugar
4 cups unbleached all-purpose flour

Directions

Preheat oven to 375 degrees F (190 degrees C). Lightly spray two 8x4x2 inch loaf pans with a non-stick cooking spray.

Combine the fat free sour cream, egg whites, vanilla, bananas and margarine and mix on medium speed of electric mixer until smooth, creamy and well blended.

Sift the flour, baking powder, baking soda, salt and light brown sugar into the banana mixture. Stir with a spoon until combined. Add more flour if necessary until a thick and rather resistant dough is formed. Fold in the optional nuts and raisins. Mix for 1 minute on the low speed of an electric mixer. Divide dough evenly between the two loaf pans.

Bake at 375 degrees F (190 degrees C) until golden and the center tests done. Remove breads from pans immediately and allow to cool on a rack before slicing.

Sweet Banana Bread

Ingredients

1 3/4 cups all-purpose flour
1 1/4 teaspoons baking powder
1/2 teaspoon baking soda
3/4 teaspoon salt
1 (3 ounce) package non-instant vanilla pudding mix
2/3 cup white sugar
1/2 cup shortening
2 eggs
2 tablespoons milk
1 1/3 cups mashed ripe banana
1/3 cup chopped walnuts

Directions

In a small bowl, sift together flour, baking powder, baking soda, salt and vanilla pudding mix. In a large mixing bowl, beat sugar and shortening until light, scraping sides of the bowl often. Add the eggs one at a time, beating smooth after each addition. Mix in the milk.

Add flour mixture and mashed bananas alternately to creamed mixture, beating until smooth after each addition. Fold in nuts if desired. Pour batter into a lightly greased 8x4 inch loaf pan.

Bake in a cold, (non-preheated) oven set to 350 degrees F (175 degrees C). Bake for 50 minutes, then cover with foil to prevent burning and bake for additional 10 to 20 minutes or until toothpick inserted into the crown comes out clean. Leave in pan for 10 minutes, then remove from pan and cool.

Strawberry Banana Protein Smoothie

Ingredients

1 banana
1 1/4 cups sliced fresh
strawberries
10 whole almonds
2 tablespoons water
1 cup ice cubes
3 tablespoons chocolate flavored
protein powder

Directions

Place the banana, strawberries, almonds, and water into a blender. Blend to mix, then add the ice cubes and puree until smooth. Add the protein powder, and continue mixing until evenly incorporated, about 30 seconds.

Banana Nut Quesadilla Wedges

Ingredients

1 tablespoon granulated sugar
1/8 teaspoon ground cinnamon
2 (8 inch) flour tortillas
Vegetable oil spread or margarine
1/4 cup JIF® Creamy Reduced Fat Peanut Spread
1 large banana, peeled and sliced 1/4-inch thick
1 tablespoon brown sugar

Directions

Combine the cinnamon and sugar. Set aside.

Cover one side of tortilla sparingly with vegetable oil spread. Place spread side down in 10-inch skillet. Spread topside with peanut butter, top with banana slices, sprinkle with brown sugar and top with remaining tortilla. Spread top of tortilla sparingly with vegetable oil spread and sprinkle with half of the cinnamon and sugar mixture.

Cover skillet. Cook over medium-high heat until the bottom is golden brown. Turn tortilla with a wide spatula. Sprinkle top with remaining cinnamon and sugar. Continue cooking covered until bottom is golden brown. Remove to cutting board and slice into 8 wedges. Serve warm.

Jif® Peanut Butter Banana Bread

Ingredients

2 1/2 cups PILLSBURY BEST® All Purpose Flour
1 cup granulated sugar
3 1/2 teaspoons baking powder
1 teaspoon salt
1 cup mashed ripe bananas 3/4 cup JIF® Crunchy Reduced Fat Peanut Spread
3/4 cup milk
1/4 cup CRISCO® Canola Oil
1 large egg

Directions

Heat oven to 350 degrees F. Grease 9 x 5 x 3-inch loaf pan.

Combine flour, sugar, baking powder and salt in large bowl. Add banana, peanut butter, milk, canola oil and egg. Beat at medium speed of electric mixer, scraping sides and bottom of bowl. Mix just until blended.

Bake at 350 degrees F for 60 to 65 minutes or until toothpick inserted in center comes out clean. (Cover top loosely with foil after 45 minutes to prevent over-browning.)

Cool 10 minutes in pan. Remove to cooling rack.

Sweetened Bananas in Coconut Milk

Ingredients

4 large bananas, cut in half
crosswise then lengthwise
1 cup coconut milk
1 cup white sugar
1 teaspoon salt
1/2 cup cream of coconut

Directions

Bring the coconut milk to a boil in a pot. Add the bananas to the coconut milk and cook until tender, about 15 minutes. Dissolve the sugar and salt into the mixture. Stir the coconut cream through the mixture. Remove from heat; serve hot.

Peanut Banana Muffins

Ingredients

1 1/2 cups all-purpose flour
1/2 cup sugar
1 teaspoon baking powder
1/2 teaspoon baking soda
1/2 teaspoon salt
1 egg
1/2 cup butter or margarine, melted
1 1/2 cups mashed ripe banana
3/4 cup peanut butter chips

Directions

In a bowl, combine the flour, sugar, baking powder, baking soda and salt. In another bowl, combine the egg, butter and bananas. Stir into dry ingredients just until moistened. Fold in chips. Fill greased or paper-lined muffin cups three-fourths full. Bake at 375 degrees F for 18-22 minutes or until toothpick comes out clean. Cool for 5 minutes before removing from pan to a wire rack.

Banana Bread French Toast

Ingredients

3 eggs
3 tablespoons sweetened condensed milk
1 teaspoon vanilla extract
2 tablespoons butter
1 loaf banana bread
confectioners' sugar for dusting (optional)

Directions

In a shallow bowl, whisk together the eggs, sweetened condensed milk and vanilla with a fork. Set aside.

Melt butter in a large skillet over medium heat. Slice banana bread into 4 thick slices. Dip each slice into the egg mixture, then place in the hot pan. Cook on each side until golden brown. Dust with confectioners' sugar just before serving, if desired.

Dietetic Banana Nut Muffins

Ingredients

1 cup all-purpose flour
1/2 cup whole wheat flour
3/4 cup granular sucrolose
sweetener (such as SplendaB®)
1 1/4 teaspoons baking powder
1 teaspoon baking soda
1 teaspoon ground cinnamon
2 egg whites
1 cup mashed ripe banana
1/4 cup applesauce

Directions

Preheat the oven to 375 degrees F (190 degrees C). Grease a 12 cup muffin tin, or line with paper muffin liners.

In a large bowl, stir together the flour, sugar substitute, baking powder, baking soda, and cinnamon. In a separate bowl, mix together the egg whites, mashed banana and applesauce. Add the wet ingredients to the dry, and mix until just blended. Fill prepared muffin cups 3/4 full.

Bake for 15 to 18 minutes in the preheated oven, or until the top springs back when lightly touched. Allow muffins to cool in the pan over a wire rack for a little while before tapping them out of the pan.

Blueberry, Banana, and Peanut Butter Smoothie

Ingredients

1 tablespoon flax seed meal or
wheat germ
1 banana
1/2 cup frozen blueberries
1 tablespoon peanut butter
1 teaspoon honey
1/2 cup plain yogurt
1 cup milk

Directions

Put ground flax seed meal or wheat germ into blender to grind and
further breakdown. This will also eliminate any bitterness from the
flax seed.

Place the banana, blueberries, peanut butter, honey, yogurt, and
milk into the blender. Cover, and puree until smooth. Pour into
glasses to serve.

Banana Dogs

Ingredients

2 tablespoons peanut butter
2 whole wheat hot dog buns
2 bananas
2 tablespoons raspberry jelly
1 tablespoon raisins (optional)

Directions

Spread 1 tablespoon of peanut butter onto each hot dog bun. Place a banana into each one as if it were a hot dog. Squeeze jelly over the banana from a squeeze bottle, or spread over the peanut butter. Sprinkle with raisins, if using.

No-Bake Mile-High Banana Split Pie

Ingredients

1 (5 ounce) package instant vanilla pudding mix
1 1/4 cups cold milk
1 (12 ounce) container frozen whipped topping, thawed, divided
2 bananas, sliced into 1/4 inch slices
1 (9 inch) prepared chocolate crumb crust
1 (12 ounce) jar hot fudge topping
2 tablespoons dark rum
1 (20 ounce) can pineapple chunks, drained
12 maraschino cherries with stems, drained
3 tablespoons walnut pieces

Directions

In a large bowl, whisk together pudding mix and milk until smooth. Fold in 2 cups of the whipped topping, and sliced banana. Reserve 1/2 of banana pudding mixture, and spread the remainder into pie crust.

In a small bowl, stir together hot fudge sauce and rum. Reserve 3 tablespoons in a microwave-safe container, for drizzling on top. With the back of a spoon, gently spread 1/2 of remaining fudge sauce over banana pudding in pie crust. Repeat layers with remaining banana pudding and remaining fudge sauce. Refrigerate for 1 hour, or until firm.

Arrange pineapple chunks in a single layer over top of pie. Spread with remaining whipped topping, swirling topping into peaks with the back of a spoon. Refrigerate for 30 minutes.

In a microwave oven, heat reserved fudge sauce until pourable, about 10 seconds. Drizzle sauce with a fork over top of pie. Garnish with maraschino cherries and chopped walnuts.

Microwave Tofu Banana Bread

Ingredients

1/2 (12 ounce) package silken tofu
2 ripe bananas
2 tablespoons miniature chocolate chips
1 cup pancake mix

Directions

Place the tofu, bananas, and 1 tablespoon of chocolate chips in the bowl of a food processor; blend on low to combine ingredients.

Mix together the pancake mix and the remaining 1 tablespoon of chocolate chips in a bowl. Stir in the banana mixture and blend until smooth. Spoon the batter into the bottom of a microwave-safe baking dish, spreading to 1 1/2 inch thickness.

Cover and cook in the microwave at full power for 3 minutes. Remove and invert onto a microwave-safe plate. If the cake is too moist, cook in the microwave 1 to 3 minutes more.

Banana Split Cake

Ingredients

1 1/2 cups HONEY MAID Graham
Cracker Crumbs
1 cup sugar, divided
1/3 cup butter, melted
2 (8 ounce) packages
PHILADELPHIA Cream Cheese,
softened
1 (20 ounce) can crushed
pineapple, drained
6 medium bananas, divided
2 cups cold milk
2 pkg. (4 serving size) JELL-O
Vanilla Flavor Instant Pudding &
Pie Filling
2 cups thawed COOL WHIP
Whipped Topping, divided
1 cup PLANTERS Chopped
Pecans

Directions

Mix crumbs, 1/4 cup of the sugar and the butter; press firmly onto bottom of 13x9-inch pan. Freeze 10 min.

Beat cream cheese and remaining 3/4 cup sugar with electric mixer on medium speed until well blended. Spread carefully over crust; top with pineapple. Slice 4 of the bananas; arrange over pineapple.

Pour milk into medium bowl. Add dry pudding mixes. Beat with wire whisk 2 min. or until well blended. Gently stir in 1 cup of the whipped topping; spread over banana layer in pan. Top with remaining 1 cup whipped topping; sprinkle with pecans. Refrigerate 5 hours. Slice remaining 2 bananas just before serving; arrange over dessert. Store leftover dessert in refrigerator.

Banana Ice Cream Shake

Ingredients

1 banana, peeled and chopped
2 scoops vanilla ice cream
1 cup milk
2 egg white
1 teaspoon vanilla extract

Directions

In a blender, combine banana, ice cream, milk, egg white and vanilla extract. Blend until smooth. Pour into glasses and serve.

Banana Caramel Fluff

Ingredients

2 bananas, peeled and sliced
1 tablespoon vanilla extract
2 tablespoons butter, melted
1 (8 ounce) can refrigerated
crescent rolls
1 cup caramel topping

Directions

Preheat oven to 350 degrees F (175 degrees C).

In a small bowl, combine bananas, vanilla and melted butter, until bananas are well coated. On a cookie sheet, unroll two crescent rolls, leaving the two triangles attached to form a square. Place 1/4 of banana mixture in the center of each pair of rolls.

Bake for 11 to 13 minutes, or until pastry is golden brown. Heat caramel topping and drizzle over dessert. Serve warm.

Banana Cranberry Muffins

Ingredients

2 cups fresh or frozen cranberries
1 2/3 cups sugar, divided
1 cup water
1/3 cup shortening
2 eggs
1 3/4 cups all-purpose flour
2 teaspoons baking powder
1/2 teaspoon salt
1/4 teaspoon baking soda
1 cup mashed ripe banana
1/2 cup chopped walnuts

Directions

In a small saucepan, bring cranberries, 1 cup sugar and water to a boil. Reduce heat; simmer, uncovered, for 5-7 minutes or until berries begin to pop. Drain and set aside.

In a large mixing bowl, cream shortening and remaining sugar. Add eggs, one at a time, beating well after each addition. Combine the flour, baking powder, salt and baking soda; add to creamed mixture alternately with bananas. Fold in cranberry mixture and walnuts.

Fill greased or paper-lined muffin cups three-fourths full. Bake at 400 degrees F for 15-20 minutes or until a toothpick comes out clean. Cool for 5 minutes before removing from pans to wire racks.

Oz's Banana-Nut and Raisin Bread for ABM

Ingredients

1 cup milk, room temperature
2 tablespoons butter, softened
2 ripe bananas
3 1/2 cups all-purpose flour
2 tablespoons white sugar
1 teaspoon salt
1 teaspoon ground cinnamon
2 1/2 teaspoons active dry yeast
or bread machine yeast
1/2 cup raisins
1/2 cup walnuts

Directions

Place the milk, butter, bananas, flour, sugar, salt, cinnamon, and yeast in the bread machine in the order recommended by the manufacturer. Select Basic setting; press Start. If your machine has a Fruit/Nut setting, add the raisins and walnuts at the signal, or around 5 minutes before the kneading cycle has finished.

Chocolate Chip Banana Muffins

Ingredients

1 1/2 cups mashed bananas
2/3 cup sunflower seed oil
1 egg, beaten
1 1/2 teaspoons vanilla extract
2 cups all-purpose flour
1/2 cup white sugar
2 tablespoons unsweetened cocoa powder
1 tablespoon baking powder
1/2 teaspoon salt
1 cup semisweet chocolate chips

Directions

Preheat oven to 425 degrees F (220 degrees C). Lightly grease a 12-cup muffin tin.

In a medium bowl blend the banana, oil, egg and vanilla together.

In a large bowl, combine the flour, sugar, cocoa, baking powder and salt. Stir in the banana mixture until just blended. Fold in the chocolate chips. Spoon the batter into the prepared muffin tin, filling 3/4 full.

Bake in the preheated oven for 15 to 20 minutes. Remove muffins to a wire rack to cool completely.

Banana Pudding V

Ingredients

1 (8 ounce) package lowfat cream cheese, softened
1 (8 ounce) container lite sour cream
1 (8 ounce) container lite frozen whipped topping, thawed
1 teaspoon vanilla extract
3 (1 ounce) packages instant sugar-free vanilla pudding mix
1/2 packet artificial sweetener
5 cups nonfat milk
1 (11 ounce) package Cookies, vanilla wafers, lower fat
7 bananas, sliced

Directions

In a medium bowl, beat cream cheese with sour cream. Stir in whipped topping and vanilla. Set aside.

In a large bowl, combine pudding mix, sweetener and milk. Stir until sugar and mix are dissolved. Combine with cheese mixture.

In a large glass serving dish, layer pudding mixture, wafers and bananas until all ingredients are used. Chill until serving.

Raspberry Banana Bread

Ingredients

1 3/4 cups all-purpose flour
1 1/2 cups sugar
1 teaspoon baking soda
1 teaspoon salt
2 eggs
1 cup mashed ripe bananas
1/2 cup vegetable oil
1/3 cup water
1 cup fresh or frozen
unsweetened raspberries*
1/2 cup chopped walnuts

Directions

In a large bowl, combine the flour, sugar, baking soda and salt. In another bowl, combine the eggs, bananas, oil and water. Stir into the dry ingredients just until moistened. Fold in raspberries and walnuts. Pour into two greased 8-in. x 4-in. x 2-in. loaf pans. Bake at 350 degrees F for 55-65 minutes or until a toothpick comes out clean. Cool for 10 minutes before removing from pans to wire racks.

Banana Split Pudding

Ingredients

3 cups cold milk
1 (5 ounce) package instant vanilla pudding mix
1 medium firm banana, sliced
1 cup sliced fresh strawberries
1 (8 ounce) can crushed pineapple, drained
1 (8 ounce) container frozen whipped topping, thawed 1/4 cup chocolate syrup
1/4 cup chopped pecans
additional sliced strawberries and bananas (optional)

Directions

In a bowl, whisk milk and pudding mix for 2 minutes. Add banana, strawberries and pineapple; transfer to a serving bowl. Dollop with whipped topping. Drizzle with chocolate syrup; sprinkle with pecans. Top with strawberries and bananas if desired.

Banana Split Cake VI

Ingredients

2 cups cornflakes cereal crumbs
1/2 cup margarine, softened

2 eggs
1 tablespoon vanilla extract
1 cup margarine
2 cups confectioners' sugar
6 banana
2 (15 ounce) cans crushed
pineapple, drained
1 (16 ounce) container frozen
whipped topping, thawed
chopped walnuts

Directions

Combine 1/2 cup margarine with cornflake crumbs, then press into the bottom of a 13x9 inch pan. Chill in the refrigerator for 30 minutes.

Mix together eggs, vanilla extract, 1 cup margarine and confectioners' sugar until smooth. Pour mixture over the chilled cornflake crust. Slice bananas lengthwise and place over the egg mixture. Spoon pineapple over the bananas, then spread whipped topping over the top to cover. Sprinkle with chopped nuts. Refrigerate overnight before serving.

Banana Bread VII

Ingredients

1/3 cup vegetable oil
1 1/2 cups mashed bananas
1/2 teaspoon vanilla extract
3 eggs
2 1/3 cups baking mix
1 cup white sugar
1/2 cup chopped walnuts

Directions

Preheat oven to 350 degrees F (175 degrees C). Generously grease the bottom of a 9 x 5 inch loaf pan.

Measure oil, bananas, vanilla, eggs, baking mix, sugar, and nuts into a large bowl. Beat vigorously with a spoon for about 30 seconds. Pour the batter into the prepared pan.

Bake until a wooden pick inserted in center comes out clean, about 55 to 65 minutes. Cool for 5 minutes in the pan. Loosen sides of loaf from the pan. Remove to a wire rack to cool completely.

Old-Fashioned Banana Cake

Ingredients

3 cups all-purpose flour
2 cups sugar
3 teaspoons baking powder
1 teaspoon salt
1 teaspoon ground cinnamon
1/4 teaspoon baking soda
3 eggs, lightly beaten
1 1/2 cups canola oil
1 1/2 teaspoons vanilla extract
1 (8 ounce) can unsweetened crushed pineapple, undrained
2 cups banana, diced
1 (10 ounce) jar maraschino cherries, drained
1 cup chopped walnuts
1 1/2 teaspoons confectioners' sugar

Directions

In a large mixing bowl, combine the first six ingredients. In a small bowl, combine the eggs, oil and vanilla. Beat into dry ingredients just until combined (batter will be thick). Stir in pineapple. Fold in the bananas, cherries and walnuts.

Transfer to a greased and floured 10-in. fluted tube pan. Bake at 350 degrees F for 60-70 minutes or until a toothpick inserted near the center comes out clean. Cool for 10 minutes before removing from pan to a wire rack to cool completely. Dust with confectioners' sugar.

Bananas Foster Belgian Waffles

Ingredients

1 1/3 cups all-purpose flour
3/4 teaspoon baking soda
2 teaspoons white sugar
1/4 teaspoon salt
3 eggs
1 1/2 teaspoons vanilla extract
1 1/3 cups milk
1/3 cup melted butter
2 teaspoons baking powder
1/4 cup butter
2/3 cup brown sugar
2 teaspoons rum flavored extract
2 teaspoons vanilla extract 1/2
teaspoon ground cinnamon 1/4
cup whole pecans
1/2 cup pancake syrup (i.e. Mrs.
Butterworth's®)
3 bananas, cut into 1/2 inch slices
1 cup heavy cream
1/4 teaspoon vanilla extract
1 tablespoon confectioners' sugar

Directions

Preheat a Belgium waffle iron. Whisk together the flour, baking soda, baking powder, white sugar, and salt in a bowl; set aside.

Whisk together the eggs, 1 1/2 teaspoons vanilla extract, and milk in a bowl. Stir in the melted butter and flour mixture until a slightly lumpy batter forms. Cook the waffles in the preheated iron until steam stops coming out of the seam, about 2 minutes.

Meanwhile, melt 1/4 cup of butter in a saucepan over medium heat. Stir in the brown sugar, rum extract, 2 teaspoons vanilla extract, and cinnamon. Bring to a simmer, the stir in the pecans and continue simmering for 1 minute. Stir in the pancake syrup and bananas, continue cooking until the bananas soften, about 4 minutes.

Beat the heavy cream, 1/4 teaspoon of vanilla and confectioners' sugar with an electric mixer in a medium bowl until firm peaks form.

Once waffles are done, spoon bananas Foster sauce over waffle and top with a dollop of whip cream.

Caramel Banana Cake Roll

Ingredients

1 cup cake flour
1/2 teaspoon baking soda
1/2 teaspoon salt
1/4 teaspoon baking powder
2 eggs
3/4 cup sugar, divided
1/2 cup mashed ripe banana
1 teaspoon vanilla extract
1 teaspoon grated lemon peel
3 egg whites
1 tablespoon confectioners' sugar
FILLING:
4 ounces reduced fat cream cheese
1/2 cup packed brown sugar
1/2 teaspoon vanilla extract
1 cup reduced-fat whipped topping
1 tablespoon confectioners' sugar
2 tablespoons fat-free caramel ice cream topping

Directions

Line a 15-in. x 10-in. x 1-in. baking pan coated with nonstick cooking spray with waxed paper and coat the paper with nonstick cooking spray; set aside.

Combine the flour, baking soda, salt and baking powder. In a large mixing bowl, beat eggs for 5 minutes; add 1/2 cup sugar, banana, vanilla and lemon peel. In a small mixing bowl, beat egg whites on medium speed until soft peaks form. Gradually beat in remaining sugar, a tablespoon at a time, on high until stiff peaks form. Add flour mixture to banana mixture; mix gently until combined. Fold in egg white mixture.

Spread into prepared pan. Bake at 375 degrees F for 10-12 minutes or until cake springs back when lightly touched. Cool for 5 minutes. Turn cake onto a kitchen towel dusted with confectioners' sugar. Gently peel off waxed paper. Roll up cake in towel jelly-roll style, starting with a short side. Cool completely on a wire rack.

For filling, in a mixing bowl, beat cream cheese and brown sugar until smooth and sugar is dissolved. Beat in vanilla; fold in whipped topping. Unroll cake; spread filling over cake to within 1/2 in. of edges. Roll up again; place seam side down on a serving platter. Cover and refrigerate for at least 1 hour before serving. Before serving, sprinkle with confectioners' sugar, then drizzle with ice cream topping. Refrigerate leftovers.

Fried Banana Dessert

Ingredients

1/2 cup semi-sweet chocolate chips
1/3 cup whipping cream
1/2 teaspoon vanilla extract
1/2 cup Cointreau or triple sec
1 tablespoon butter
6 bananas, peeled and halved lengthwise
1 cup toasted sliced almonds

Directions

Place chocolate chips, cream, and vanilla extract into a small saucepan. Stir over medium-low heat until the chocolate chips have melted. Stir in the Cointreau and set aside.

Melt butter in a large skillet over medium-high heat. Add bananas, cut-side down, and cook until golden brown, 3 to 4 minutes. Turn bananas over, and continue cooking until golden brown on the other side, 3 to 4 minutes more.

To serve, ladle some of the sauce onto the center of 6 plates. Place two banana halves onto each plate, and sprinkle with toasted almonds.

Banana Split Salad

Ingredients

1 (14 ounce) can sweetened condensed milk
1 (12 ounce) container frozen whipped topping, thawed
1 (21 ounce) can cherry pie filling
3 medium firm bananas, cut into chunks
1 (8 ounce) can crushed pineapple, drained
1/2 cup chopped nuts

Directions

In a large bowl, combine the milk and whipped topping until well blended. Fold in pie filling, bananas, pineapple and nuts.

Emily's Famous Banana Oat Muffins

Ingredients

3 ripe bananas, mashed
1 cup brown sugar
1 egg
1 teaspoon vanilla extract
1/2 cup vegetable oil
2 cups whole wheat flour
1 cup rolled oats
1/2 teaspoon ground cinnamon
1/2 teaspoon ginger
1 tablespoon baking powder
1/2 teaspoon baking soda

Directions

Preheat the oven to 350 degrees F (175 degrees C). Line a 12 cup muffin pan with paper liners or coat with cooking spray.

In a large bowl, stir together the bananas, brown sugar, egg, vanilla and oil. Combine the whole wheat flour, oats, cinnamon, ginger, baking powder and baking soda; stir into the banana mixture until blended. Spoon the batter into the prepared muffin cups.

Bake in the preheated oven until the tops spring back when lightly pressed, about 25 minutes. Cool for a few minutes in the pan before attempting to remove them.

Chocolate-Banana Shake

Ingredients

1 banana
1 3/4 cups milk
3 tablespoons powdered chocolate drink mix
2 tablespoons SPLENDA® No Calorie Sweetener, Granulated

Directions

In a blender, combine banana, milk, chocolate drink mix and SPLENDA® Granulated Sweetener. Blend until smooth. Pour into glasses and serve.

Banana Butter Icing

Ingredients

1/4 cup butter, softened
1/2 cup mashed bananas
1/2 teaspoon lemon juice
1/2 teaspoon vanilla extract
3 1/4 cups confectioners' sugar

Directions

Cream together butter, banana, lemon juice and vanilla. Slowly beat in confectioners' sugar, adding more if needed to make a nice fluffy, spreadable icing. Makes about 2 1/3 cups.

Favorite Banana Blueberry Quick Bread

Ingredients

1/2 cup fresh blueberries
1 5/8 cups all-purpose flour
1/2 cup quick cooking oats
1/2 cup chopped pecans
1 teaspoon baking soda
1/4 teaspoon salt
1/2 cup shortening
1 cup white sugar
2 eggs
1 cup mashed bananas

Directions

Preheat oven to 350 degrees F (175 degrees C). Grease and flour a 9x5 inch loaf pan.

In a medium bowl, dredge blueberries in 2 tablespoons flour. Gently stir blueberries together with oats, nuts, 1 1/2 cups flour, soda, and salt.

In a large bowl, cream shortening. Gradually add sugar, beating until light and fluffy. Add eggs one at a time, beating well after each addition. Stir in mashed banana. Add blueberry mixture to creamed mixture, and stir just until moistened. Spoon batter into the prepared pan.

Bake for 50 to 55 minutes, or until a wooden toothpick comes out clean when inserted in the center of the loaf. Cool in pan for 10 minutes. Remove from pan, and cool completely on a wire rack.

Strawberry Banana Pie

Ingredients

1 unbaked pie crust
1/2 cup cold butter, cut into small pieces
1/4 cup packed brown sugar
1 cup all-purpose flour
1 tablespoon ground cinnamon
1 tablespoon ground nutmeg
2 tablespoons chopped walnuts (optional)
1/4 cup apple juice
3 ripe bananas, sliced
1/4 cup honey
1 cup chopped fresh strawberries
1/2 cup white sugar

Directions

Preheat oven to 375 degrees F (190 degrees C). Press the prepared pie crust into a 9 inch pie pan and set aside.

Combine the butter, brown sugar, flour, cinnamon, nutmeg, and nuts in the bowl of a food processor. Pulse the mixture until it has the texture of oatmeal. Refrigerate this crumble topping until ready to use.

Pour the apple juice into a medium sauce pan over medium-low heat; add the sliced bananas and honey and stir until the honey melts. Mix in the chopped strawberries and white sugar. Simmer uncovered for 20 minutes. Pour the warm fruit mixture into the prepared pie crust; evenly distribute the cold crumble topping across the top of the pie.

Bake in the preheated oven until golden brown and set, about 20 minutes. Cool the pie on a wire rack for 30 minutes before serving.

Gritty Banana Mango Corn Muffins

Ingredients

1 cup cornmeal
1 cup couscous
3 tablespoons brown sugar
1 teaspoon baking powder
1 teaspoon baking soda
1/2 teaspoon salt
1/2 cup chopped dried mango
2 very ripe bananas, mashed
2 eggs
1/4 cup vegetable oil
1 teaspoon vanilla extract
1 cup buttermilk

Directions

Preheat oven to 400 degrees F (200 degrees C). Whisk together the cornmeal, couscous, brown sugar, baking powder, baking soda, and salt in a bowl. Stir in the dried mango.

Whisk together the mashed bananas, eggs, vegetable oil, vanilla extract, and buttermilk. Stir the cornmeal mixture into the banana mixture, and let the batter rest until the couscous absorbs some of the moisture, about 5 minutes. Spoon the batter into ungreased muffin cups, filling them 2/3 full.

Bake in the preheated oven until lightly browned, and a toothpick inserted into the center comes out clean, about 15 minutes. Cool in the pans for 10 minutes before removing. Serve warm or at room temperature.

Chocolate Banana Bread

Ingredients

1 cup margarine, softened
2 cups white sugar
4 eggs
6 bananas, mashed
2 teaspoons vanilla extract
3 cups all-purpose flour
2 teaspoons baking soda
1/4 cup unsweetened cocoa powder
1 cup lite sour cream
1 cup semisweet chocolate chips

Directions

Preheat oven to 350 degrees F (175 degrees C). Lightly grease two 9x5 inch loaf pans.

In a large bowl, cream together margarine, sugar and eggs. Stir in bananas and vanilla. Sift in flour, baking soda and cocoa; mix well. Blend in sour cream and chocolate chips. Pour batter into prepared pans.

Bake in preheated oven for 60 minutes, or until a toothpick inserted into center of a loaf comes out clean.

Mimi's Giant Whole-Wheat Banana-Strawberry

Ingredients

2 eggs
1/2 cup unsweetened applesauce
1/4 cup vegetable oil
3/4 cup packed brown sugar
1 teaspoon vanilla extract
3 bananas, mashed
2 cups whole wheat flour
1 teaspoon baking soda
1 tablespoon ground cinnamon
1 cup frozen sliced strawberries

Directions

Preheat the oven to 375 degrees F (190 degrees C). Grease 12 large muffin cups, or line with paper liners.

In a large bowl, whisk together the eggs, applesauce, oil, brown sugar, vanilla and bananas. Combine the flour, baking soda and cinnamon; Stir into the banana mixture until moistened. Stir in the strawberries until evenly distributed. Spoon batter into muffin cups until completely filled.

Bake for 20 minutes in the preheated oven, or until the tops of the muffins spring back when pressed lightly. Cool before removing from the muffin tins.

Brazilian Whole Banana Pie

Ingredients

3 tablespoons brown sugar
1/2 cup water
10 bananas, peeled and sliced lengthwise
2 cups whole wheat flour
2 cups toasted wheat germ
3 cups rolled oats
1 cup packed brown sugar
1 cup light margarine
1 tablespoon cinnamon

Directions

Preheat the oven to 350 degrees F (175 degrees C).

Sprinkle 3 tablespoons of brown sugar over the bottom of a small saucepan or skillet. Cook over medium heat until melted. Stir in water until sugar is completely dissolved. Heat to between 234 and 240 degrees F (112 to 116 degrees C), or until a small amount of syrup dropped into cold water forms a soft ball that flattens when removed from the water and placed on a flat surface. Pour the syrup into a round baking dish or deep dish pie plate and spread to coat the bottom.

Make a layer of bananas on top of the melted sugar. In a medium bowl, stir together the whole wheat flour, wheat germ, oats and 1 cup of brown sugar. Mix in the margarine using your hands, pinching it into small pieces to make a crumbly dough. Sprinkle half of this over the bananas in the dish and pat down. Top with the remaining bananas and sprinkle with about half of the cinnamon. Spread the rest of the dough over the bananas and pat the pie smooth. Sprinkle remaining cinnamon over the top.

Bake for 45 minutes in the preheated oven, until the pie topping is toasted and a toothpick inserted into the center comes out clean.

Strawberry Banana Blend

Ingredients

2 bananas, sliced
15 strawberries, hulled
1/2 cup fresh peaches, pitted and chopped
1 3/4 cups strawberry sorbet
1/3 cup orange juice

Directions

In a blender combine the bananas and strawberries. Blend on medium speed until smooth. Blend in the peaches and orange juice. Scoop in the sorbet. Blend until smooth.

Banana Cream Pie with Caramel Drizzle

Ingredients

1 medium banana, sliced
1 (6 ounce) HONEY MAID Graham Pie Crust
2 cups cold milk
2 pkg. (4 serving size) JELL-O Vanilla Flavor Instant Pudding & Pie Filling
2 cups thawed COOL WHIP French Vanilla Whipped Topping, divided
1/4 cup KRAFT Caramel Topping

Directions

Arrange banana slices on bottom of crust.

Pour milk into large bowl. Add dry pudding mixes. Beat with wire whisk 2 min. or until well blended. Gently stir in 1 cup of the whipped topping; spoon into crust.

Refrigerate 4 hours or until set. Top with remaining 1 cup whipped topping just before serving. Drizzle with caramel topping. Store leftover pie in refrigerator.

Banana Butterscotch Bread

Ingredients

2 cups all-purpose flour
1 teaspoon baking powder
1/2 teaspoon baking soda
1/2 teaspoon salt
3/4 teaspoon ground cinnamon
1/2 teaspoon ground nutmeg 1/2
cup butter
3/4 cup white sugar
1 large egg
3 ripe bananas, mashed
3/4 cup butterscotch chips
1/2 cup chopped walnuts
(optional)

Directions

Preheat an oven to 350 degrees F (175 degrees C). Grease 2 9x5-inch loaf pans. Set aside. Sift the flour, baking powder, baking soda, salt, cinnamon, and nutmeg together in a bowl. Set aside.

Beat the butter and sugar with an electric mixer in a large bowl until light and fluffy. The mixture should be noticeably lighter in color. Beat in the egg, then stir in the mashed bananas. Pour in the flour mixture, mixing until just incorporated. Fold in the butterscotch chips and walnuts; mixing just enough to evenly combine. Pour the batter evenly into the prepared pans.

Bake in the preheated oven until a toothpick inserted into the center comes out clean, 25 to 28 minutes. Cool in the pans for 10 minutes before removing to cool completely on a wire rack.

Banana Streusel Muffins

Ingredients

2 cups all-purpose flour
1 cup sugar
1 teaspoon baking powder
1/2 teaspoon salt
1/2 teaspoon baking soda
1/4 teaspoon ground cinnamon
2 eggs
1 cup sour cream
1/4 cup butter or margarine, melted
2 medium ripe bananas, mashed
STREUSEL:
1/4 cup sugar
3 tablespoons all-purpose flour
1/4 teaspoon ground cinnamon
2 tablespoons butter or margarine

Directions

In a large bowl, combine the flour, sugar, baking powder, salt, baking soda and cinnamon. In a small bowl, beat eggs, sour cream, butter and bananas; stir into dry ingredients just until moistened. Fill greased or paper-lined muffin cups three-fourths full.

For streusel, combine sugar, flour and cinnamon in a small bowl; cut in butter. Sprinkle over muffins. Bake at 375 degrees F for 20-25 minutes.

Oatmeal Banana Nut Bread

Ingredients

1/2 cup shortening
3/4 cup white sugar
2 eggs
1 cup mashed bananas
1 teaspoon vanilla extract
1 1/2 cups all-purpose flour
1/2 teaspoon baking soda
1/2 teaspoon salt
1/2 cup quick cooking oats
1/2 cup chopped walnuts

Directions

Preheat oven to 350 degrees F (175 degrees C). Lightly grease a 9x5 inch loaf pan.

In a large bowl, cream together the shortening and sugar until light and fluffy. Stir in the eggs one at a time, beating well with each addition, then stir in the banana and vanilla.

In a separate bowl, sift together flour, baking soda and salt. Beat into creamed mixture. Stir in oats and nuts. Pour into prepared pan.

Bake in preheated oven for 50 to 55 minutes, or until a toothpick inserted into the center of the loaf comes out clean.

Healthy Banana Cookies

Ingredients

3 ripe bananas
2 cups rolled oats
1 cup dates, pitted and chopped
1/3 cup vegetable oil
1 teaspoon vanilla extract

Directions

Preheat oven to 350 degrees F (175 degrees C).

In a large bowl, mash the bananas. Stir in oats, dates, oil, and vanilla. Mix well, and allow to sit for 15 minutes. Drop by teaspoonfuls onto an ungreased cookie sheet.

Bake for 20 minutes in the preheated oven, or until lightly brown.

Banana Custard Scrunch

Ingredients

1 cup plain yogurt
3/4 cup prepared vanilla pudding
3/4 cup rolled oats
2 tablespoons honey
3 small bananas, sliced

Directions

In a small bowl, stir together the yogurt and vanilla pudding. Set aside.

Heat a dry skillet over medium heat. Measure in the oats, and toast for about 1 minute, until hot. Drizzle honey over the oats, and continue to stir over medium heat until the oats are crispy at the edges.

Remove the oats from the heat, and spoon most of them into the bottom of 4 glasses or small bowls. Reserve the rest for topping. Using about half of the banana slices, place a layer of sliced bananas over the oats in each glass or bowl. Pour custard over the banana slices. Top with the rest of the banana slices, and sprinkle with the rest of the toasted oats.

Vanilla-Banana Smoothie

Ingredients

2 bananas, broken into chunks
1 cup vanilla ice cream
1/2 teaspoon vanilla extract
1/2 cup fresh orange juice
1 cup milk

Directions

Place banana and vanilla ice cream into a blender. Pour in vanilla extract, orange juice, and milk. Puree until thick and smooth.

Chocolate Banana Cream Pie

Ingredients

1 (9 inch) deep dish pie crust,
baked and cooled
2 (1 ounce) squares semisweet
chocolate
1 tablespoon milk
1 tablespoon butter
2 bananas, sliced
1 1/2 cups cold milk
1 (3.5 ounce) package instant
vanilla pudding mix
1 1/2 cups shredded coconut
1 1/2 cups frozen whipped
topping, thawed
2 tablespoons flaked coconut,
toasted

Directions

Combine chocolate, 1 tablespoon milk, and butter or margarine in a medium, microwave safe bowl. Microwave on high for 1 to 1 1/2 minutes, stirring every 30 seconds. Stir until chocolate is completely melted. Spread evenly in pie crust.

Arrange banana slices over chocolate.

Pour 1 1/2 cups milk into a large bowl. Add pudding mix, and beat with wire whisk for 2 minutes. Stir in 1 1/2 cups coconut. Spoon over banana slices in crust.

Spread whipped topping over pie. Sprinkle with toasted coconut. Refrigerate 4 hours, or until set. Store in refrigerator.

Bananas Foster II

Ingredients

1/4 cup butter
2/3 cup dark brown sugar
3 1/2 tablespoons rum
1 1/2 teaspoons vanilla extract
1/2 teaspoon ground cinnamon
3 bananas, peeled and sliced lengthwise and crosswise
1/4 cup coarsely chopped walnuts
1 pint vanilla ice cream

Directions

In a large, deep skillet over medium heat, melt butter. Stir in sugar, rum, vanilla and cinnamon. When mixture begins to bubble, place bananas and walnuts in pan. Cook until bananas are hot, 1 to 2 minutes. Serve at once over vanilla ice cream.

Banana Empanadas

Ingredients

1/4 cup raisins
2 1/2 cups all-purpose flour
1/2 teaspoon salt
3/4 cup shortening
2 tablespoons plain yogurt
1/2 cup cold water

4 large ripe bananas, coarsely chopped
1/2 teaspoon ground cinnamon, or to taste

1 tablespoon cold water
1 egg white

Directions

Soak raisins in hot water for 30 minutes. Preheat the oven to 425 degrees F (220 degrees C).

In a large bowl, mix together the flour and salt. Mix in shortening using a fork, until the entire mixture is in pea-sized pellets. Stir in yogurt, and just enough of the 1/2 cup of cold water to hold it together in a dough.

Roll out dough to a square 1/8 inch in thickness. Use a knife to cut into four 8x8 inch squares. Don't worry if they aren't perfect. Drain the raisins, and mix with the cinnamon and chopped bananas. Spoon some of the banana mixture onto half of each square, leaving at least 1/2 inch of dough exposed at the edge to seal the edges. Fold the dough over the fruit, and pinch the edges together. Make sure that they are secure. I like to roll the excess dough up around the edges and then pinch it until it's thin again. You'll want to have about a 1/2 inch closure in the end. You can trim the edges a bit to make them more aesthetically pleasing. Place empanadas on a baking sheet. Whisk together 1 tablespoon of cold water and egg white; brush over the tops.

Bake for 30 minutes in the preheated oven, or until golden brown.

Banana Chip Cookies

Ingredients

3/4 cup shortening
1 cup sugar
2 eggs
1/2 cup milk
1/4 cup honey
1 medium ripe banana, mashed
4 cups all-purpose flour
2 teaspoons baking powder
1 teaspoon salt
1 cup miniature semisweet chocolate chips

Directions

In a mixing bowl, cream shortening and sugar. Add eggs, one at a time, beating well after each addition. Beat in milk, honey and banana. Combine flour, baking powder and salt; gradually add to the creamed mixture. Stir in chocolate chips.

Drop by heaping teaspoonfuls 2 in. apart onto lightly greased baking sheets. Flatten with a glass dipped in sugar. Bake at 350 degrees F for 10-12 minutes or until edges are lightly browned. Remove to wire racks to cool.

Green Banana Fries

Ingredients

5 small unripe (green) bananas
1 quart oil for frying, or as needed
salt to taste

Directions

Peel the bananas using a knife, as they are not ripe and will not peel like a yellow banana. Slice into long thin wedges or strings to make fries.

Heat the oil in a heavy deep skillet over medium-high heat. If you have a deep-fryer, heat the oil to 375 degrees F (190 degrees C). Place the banana fries into the hot oil, and fry until golden brown, 5 to 7 minutes. Remove from the oil, and drain on paper towels. Pat off the excess oil, and season with salt. Serve immediately.

Banana Split Cake II

Ingredients

1 (16 ounce) package vanilla wafers, crushed
1 cup margarine, melted
1 (20 ounce) can crushed pineapple, drained
6 bananas
1 (8 ounce) package cream cheese
2 cups confectioners' sugar
1 (12 ounce) container frozen whipped topping, thawed
1/4 cup chopped walnuts
8 maraschino cherries

Directions

Combine the crushed vanilla wafers and melted margarine. Pat into the bottom of one 9x13 inch pan.

Beat the cream cheese and confectioners' sugar together until light and fluffy. Spread over the top of the vanilla wafer crust. Spoon crushed pineapple over the cream cheese layer. Then layer sliced bananas over the pineapple. Cover with the non-dairy whipped topping and sprinkle top with chopped walnuts and maraschino cherries.

Banana Pudding Crunch

Ingredients

2 cups cold milk
2 (3.4 ounce) packages instant vanilla pudding mix
1/2 cup sour cream
2 medium firm bananas. sliced
1 cup sugar
1 cup chopped pecans
1 egg, beaten

Directions

In a bowl, combine milk, pudding mix and sour cream; whisk until mixture begins to thicken, about 1 minute. Fold in bananas. Pour into a 1-1/2-qt. serving bowl. Cover and refrigerate.

For topping, combine sugar, pecans and egg; spoon onto a greased 15-in. x 10-in. x 1-in. baking pan. Bake at 350 degrees F for 20 minutes or until browned and crunchy. Cool. Using a spatula, loosen pecan mixture from pan and break into a small pieces. Sprinkle over pudding just before serving.

Banana Upside-Down Cake

Ingredients

4 tablespoons butter, melted
1/2 cup brown sugar
1/2 cup chopped pecans
4 bananas, sliced
1 (18.25 ounce) package banana cake mix

Directions

Preheat oven to 350 degrees F (175 degrees C). Grease and flour 2 (8 inch) pans. Combine butter and brown sugar, divide and spread evenly between the 2 pans. Sprinkle pecans evenly over both brown sugar mixtures, arrange banana slices evenly over each.

Prepare cake mix according to package instructions. Divide batter into the 2 pans.

Bake in the preheated oven for 40 to 45 minutes, or until a toothpick inserted into the center of the cake comes out clean. Turn cakes upside down on a platter or plate, gently tap bottom and carefully remove pans, replacing caramel mixture that sticks to pan.

Banana Bread V

Ingredients

2 cups all-purpose flour
1/2 teaspoon baking soda
1 cup white sugar
1 egg
5 tablespoons milk
1 teaspoon baking powder
1/2 teaspoon salt
1/2 cup margarine
1 cup mashed bananas
1/2 cup chopped walnuts
(optional)

Directions

Sift together flour, baking soda, baking powder, and salt.

In a large bowl, cream sugar and butter or margarine. Beat the egg slightly, and mix into the creamed mixture with the bananas. Mix in sifted ingredients until just combined. Stir in milk and nuts. Spread batter into one greased and floured 9x5 inch loaf pan.

Bake at 350 degrees F (175 degrees C) until top is brown and cracks along the top.

Banana Muffins with a Crunch

Ingredients

3 cups all-purpose flour
2 cups white sugar
2 teaspoons baking powder
1 teaspoon baking soda
1 teaspoon salt
2 eggs, lightly beaten
3/4 cup milk
2 teaspoons vanilla extract
1 cup melted butter, cooled
2 bananas, mashed
1 banana, chopped
1 cup granola
1 cup chopped walnuts
1 cup shredded coconut
1/4 cup banana chips (optional)

Directions

Preheat oven to 350 degrees F (175 degrees C). Line 24 muffin cups with paper liners.

In a bowl, mix the flour, sugar, baking powder, baking soda, and salt. Mix in the eggs, milk, vanilla, and butter. Fold in mashed bananas, chopped banana, granola, walnuts, and coconut. Scoop into the prepared muffin cups. Sprinkle with banana chips.

Bake 25 minutes in the preheated oven, or until a knife inserted in the center of a muffin comes out clean.

Hawaiian Banana Nut Bread

Ingredients

3 cups all-purpose flour
3/4 teaspoon salt
1 teaspoon baking soda
2 cups white sugar
1 teaspoon ground cinnamon
1 cup chopped walnuts
3 eggs, beaten
1 cup vegetable oil
2 cups mashed very ripe banana
1 (8 ounce) can crushed
pineapple, drained
2 teaspoons vanilla extract
1 cup flaked coconut
1 cup maraschino cherries, diced

Directions

Preheat oven to 350 degrees F (175 degrees C). Grease two 9x5 inch loaf pans.

In a large mixing bowl, combine the flour, salt, baking soda, sugar and cinnamon. Add the walnuts, eggs, oil, banana, pineapple, vanilla, coconut and cherries; stir just until blended. Pour batter evenly into the prepared pans.

Bake at 350 degrees F (175 degrees C) for 60 minutes, or until a tooth pick inserted into the center of a loaf comes out clean. Cool in the pan for 10 minutes, then remove to a wire rack to cool completely.

Warm Tropical Banana Ice Cream Topping

Ingredients

3 tablespoons butter
6 ripe bananas, sliced
2 teaspoons vanilla extract
1 cup sweetened flaked coconut
3 1/2 tablespoons confectioners' sugar
1/4 cup chopped walnuts

Directions

Melt the butter in a skillet over medium heat. Place the banana slices in the skillet, stir in the vanilla, and cook until bananas are golden brown. Stir in the coconut, and top with confectioners' sugar and walnuts. Serve immediately over ice cream.

Banana-Cream Cheesecake

Ingredients

1 (18.25 ounce) package white cake mix, divided
4 eggs, divided
3 tablespoons oil
2/3 cup packed brown sugar, divided
2 bananas, sliced
2 (8 ounce) packages PHILADELPHIA Cream Cheese, softened
2 tablespoons lemon juice
1 1/2 cups milk
1 1/2 cups thawed COOL WHIP Whipped Topping

Directions

Heat oven to 300 degrees F. Reserve 1 cup dry cake mix. Mix remaining cake mix with 1 egg, oil and 1/3 cup sugar with mixer. (Mixture will be crumbly.) Press onto bottom and 1 inch up sides of greased 13x9-inch baking pan; top with bananas.

Beat cream cheese and remaining sugar with mixer. Add reserved cake mix, remaining eggs and lemon juice; beat 1 minute. Blend in milk. (Batter will be very thin.) Pour into crust.

Bake 45 to 50 to minutes or until center is almost set. Cool. Refrigerate 4 hours. Top with COOL WHIP. Refrigerate leftovers.

Strawberry-Banana-Peanut Butter Smoothie

Ingredients

1/2 cup nonfat plain yogurt
2 tablespoons peanut butter
1 banana
4 fresh strawberries, hulled
10 ice cubes

Directions

Place yogurt, peanut butter, banana, strawberries, and ice cubes into a blender. Puree until smooth.

Jumbo Banana Cookies

Ingredients

1/2 cup shortening
1/2 cup butter, softened
1 cup white sugar
2 eggs
1 cup mashed bananas
1/2 cup evaporated milk
1 teaspoon vanilla extract
1 teaspoon distilled white vinegar
3 cups all-purpose flour
1 1/2 teaspoons baking soda
1/2 teaspoon salt
1 cup chopped walnuts
2 1/2 cups confectioners' sugar
2 tablespoons butter, softened
1/4 cup evaporated milk
1/4 teaspoon vanilla extract

Directions

Mix together shortening, 1/2 cup butter, white sugar, eggs, bananas, vanilla, 1/2 cup evaporated milk and vinegar till light and creamy.

In a separate bowl mix together flour, baking soda, and salt. Add to other mixture. Add nuts.

Chill one hour in refrigerator.

Drop by teaspoonful on greased cookie sheet about two inches apart. Bake at 375 degrees F (190 degrees C) for about 15 minutes. Let cool then frost them.

To Make Frosting: Mix 2 1/2 cups confectioners' sugar with 2 tablespoons soft butter or margarine, 1/4 cup evaporated milk, and 1/4 tsp vanilla. Beat until soft. Spread on tops of cooled cookies.

Joy's Green Banana Salad

Ingredients

6 small unripe (green) bananas
2 tablespoons olive oil, divided
1 green bell pepper, sliced into thin rings
1 cup small shrimp - peeled and deveined
1 cup crabmeat
1 sweet onion, chopped
1 pinch salt and pepper to taste
1 teaspoon white sugar
3/4 cup red wine vinegar
2 slices crisp cooked bacon, crumbled
1 hard-cooked egg, peeled and sliced (optional)

Directions

Bring a large pot of water to a boil. Cut the ends off of the bananas, and make a slit lengthwise down the peel. Cook bananas in boiling water until tender (similar to a potato). Drain, cool, and remove peels. Cut into small chunks and place in a serving bowl. Drizzle 1 tablespoon of olive oil over the pieces, and stir to coat.

Meanwhile, heat the remaining tablespoon of oil in a skillet over medium-high heat. Add shrimp and crab, and fry until cooked through, about 5 minutes. Set aside to cool.

Add onions, green pepper and seafood to the bananas in the bowl. In a separate bowl, whisk together the red wine vinegar, sugar and bacon pieces. Pour this mixture over the bananas, and toss lightly to coat. Season with salt and pepper. Garnish with slices of hard-cooked egg if desired.

Banana Nut Bread Baked in a Jar

Ingredients

2/3 cup shortening
2 2/3 cups white sugar
4 eggs
2 cups mashed bananas
2/3 cup water
3 1/3 cups all-purpose flour
1/2 teaspoon baking powder
2 teaspoons baking soda
1 1/2 teaspoons salt
1 teaspoon ground cinnamon
1 teaspoon ground cloves
2/3 cup chopped pecans

Directions

Preheat oven to 325 degrees F (165 degrees C). Grease insides of 8 (1 pint) straight sided, wide mouth canning jars.

In a large bowl, cream shortening and sugar until light and fluffy. Beat in eggs, bananas, and water. Sift together flour, baking powder, soda, salt, cinnamon, and cloves. Add to banana mixture. Stir in nuts.

Pour mixture into greased WIDE MOUTH pint jars, filling 1/2 full of batter. Do NOT put lids on jars for baking. Be careful to keep the rims clean, wiping off any batter that gets on the rims.

Bake at 325 degrees F (165 degrees C) for 45 minutes. Meanwhile, sterilize the lids and rings in boiling water.

As soon as cake is done, remove from oven one at a time, wipe rims of jars and put on lid and ring. Jars will seal as cakes cool. Place the jars on the counter and listen for them to "ping" as they seal. If you miss the "ping", wait until they are completely cool and press on the top of the lid. If it doesn't move at all, it's sealed.

Jars should be eaten immediately or kept sealed in refrigerator for up to a week.

Hawaiian Baked Bananas

Ingredients

4 bananas, peeled
1/2 cup brown sugar, firmly packed
1/4 cup orange or pineapple juice
3 tablespoons sherry
1 dash nutmeg
2 tablespoons butter
1/2 cup chopped almonds or macadamia nuts

Directions

Preheat oven to 350 degrees F (175 degrees C).

Place the bananas into a small glass baking dish. Stir together the brown sugar, juice, and sherry; pour over the bananas, then sprinkle with nutmeg. Melt the butter in a small pan over medium heat. Stir in chopped nuts, and cook until lightly browned, about 4 minutes. Pour over the banana mixture.

Bake in preheated oven for 15 minutes until the bananas are tender, and have become lightly glazed.

Banana Pancakes with Berries

Ingredients

2 cups sliced fresh strawberries
1/2 cup sugar
3 teaspoons vanilla extract
PANCAKES:
1 cup all-purpose flour
1 tablespoon sugar
1 teaspoon baking powder
1/2 teaspoon baking soda
1/2 teaspoon salt
1 egg
1 cup buttermilk
2 tablespoons vegetable oil
1 teaspoon vanilla extract
2 medium ripe bananas, cut into
1/4-inch slices
Whipped cream

Directions

In a bowl, combine the strawberries, sugar and vanilla. Cover and refrigerate for 8 hours or overnight.

For pancakes, combine the flour, sugar, baking powder, baking soda and salt in a bowl. Combine the egg, buttermilk, oil and vanilla; stir into dry ingredients just until moistened.

Pour the batter by 1/4 cupfuls onto a lightly greased hot griddle; place 5-6 banana slices on each pancake. Turn when bubbles form on top; cook until second side is golden brown. Serve with strawberries and whipped cream if desired.

Chocolate Banana Crepes

Ingredients

Crepe Batter:
1/2 cup whole or 2% milk
1 1/2 tablespoons melted butter
1 egg yolk
1 teaspoon vanilla
2 teaspoons hazelnut liqueur
1 tablespoon cocoa
2 tablespoons confectioners' sugar
1/3 cup white flour

Chocolate Sauce:
1/2 tablespoon butter
1 tablespoon whole or 2% milk
2 teaspoons hazelnut liqueur
1 tablespoon cocoa
2 tablespoons confectioners' sugar

2 ripe bananas, sliced

Directions

In a medium bowl, stir together 1/2 cup milk, 1 1/2 tablespoons melted butter, egg yolk, vanilla, and 2 teaspoons hazelnut liqueur. Whisk 1 tablespoon cocoa into liquid until completely incorporated. Next, whisk in 2 tablespoons confectioners' sugar until completely incorporated. Then gradually whisk in flour until completely incorporated. Set aside.

Melt 1/2 tablespoon butter in a saucepan over low heat. Stir 1 tablespoon milk and 2 teaspoons hazelnut liqueur into melted butter. Stir in 1 tablespoon cocoa and 2 tablespoons confectioners' sugar. Set over very low heat to keep warm.

Spray a non-stick frying pan or crepe pan with cooking spray, and heat over medium heat. Pour about 1/4 cup of batter onto the pan, and swirl to form a very thin disk; cook for about 2 minutes. Flip, and cook about 1 minute more.

Place crepe on a plate. Add 1/4 sliced bananas to crepe, and spoon 1/4 of the chocolate sauce over the bananas. Roll or fold crepe, and sprinkle with confectioners' sugar. Repeat steps 3 and 4. Serve crepes warm.

Banana Date Flaxseed Bread

Ingredients

1/2 cup flax seed
3 bananas, mashed
1/4 cup vegetable oil
1/2 cup white sugar
2 eggs
1 1/2 cups all-purpose flour
1/2 teaspoon baking powder
1/2 teaspoon baking soda 1/2
teaspoon salt
1/4 cup flax seed
1/2 cup chopped pitted dates

Directions

Preheat oven to 350 degrees F (175 degrees C). Lightly grease an 8x4 inch loaf pan. Use an electric coffee grinder or food processor to grind 1/2 cup flax seed; set aside.

In a large mixing bowl, beat together banana, oil, sugar and eggs. In a separate bowl, mix together flour, baking powder, baking soda, salt, ground flax seed and 1/4 cup whole flax seed. Gradually stir flour mixture into banana mixture. Fold in dates. Spoon batter into prepared loaf pan.

Bake in preheated oven for 55 to 60 minutes, or until a toothpick inserted into the loaf comes out clean.

Banana Frittata

Ingredients

1/2 cup all-purpose flour
1 pinch salt
2 tablespoons white sugar
1/4 cup milk
2 eggs
2 large bananas, sliced
2 tablespoons vegetable oil
1/2 tablespoon butter

Directions

In a bowl, combine the flour, salt and sugar. Gradually pour in the milk, stirring constantly, until a smooth batter is formed. Add the eggs, one at time, stirring well each addition. Stir in sliced bananas.

Heat oil and butter in a nine inch non-stick skillet over medium heat. Pour the mixture in by spoonfuls, spreading the mixture evenly across the pan. When the bottom has turned a golden brown turn the frittata and cook over low heat until golden brown on the other side. Sprinkle with sugar and serve warm.

Banana-Berry Brownie Pizza

Ingredients

1 (19.8 ounce) package fudge
brownie mix
1/3 cup boiling water
1/4 cup vegetable oil
1 egg
TOPPING:
1 (8 ounce) package cream
cheese, softened
1/4 cup sugar
1 egg
1 teaspoon vanilla extract
2 cups sliced fresh strawberries
1 medium firm banana, sliced
1 (1 ounce) square semisweet
chocolate, melted

Directions

In a bowl, combine the brownie mix, water, oil and egg until well
blended. Spread into a greased and floured 12-in. pizza pan. Bake at
350 degrees F for 25 minutes.

In a mixing bowl, beat the cream cheese, sugar, egg and vanilla until
combined. Spread over brownie crust. Bake 15 minutes longer or until
topping is set. Cool on a wire rack.

Just before serving, arrange strawberries and bananas over
topping; drizzle with chocolate. Refrigerate leftovers.

Banana Oatmeal Bread

Ingredients

1/2 cup shortening
1 cup white sugar
2 eggs, beaten
1/2 teaspoon vanilla extract
1 cup all-purpose flour
1 cup quick cooking oats
1 teaspoon baking soda
1/2 teaspoon salt
1/2 teaspoon ground cinnamon
1 1/2 cups mashed bananas
1/4 cup milk
1/2 cup chopped raisins (optional)

Directions

Preheat oven to 350 degrees F (175 degrees C). Grease one 9x5 inch loaf pan and set aside.

Cream together the shortening and sugar. Add eggs and vanilla, beat until fluffy.

Sift together the flour, oatmeal, baking soda, salt and cinnamon. Add dry ingredients alternately with bananas and milk. Mix until blended.

Fold in raisins and pour into prepared pan. Bake for 50 to 60 minutes; remove from oven and cover for 5 minutes.

Banana Caramel Pie II

Ingredients

1 (14 ounce) can sweetened condensed milk
3 bananas
1 (9 inch) prepared graham cracker crust
1 (12 ounce) container frozen whipped topping, thawed

Directions

Fill a saucepan with 2 inches of water. Place an unopened can of sweetened condensed milk into the water. Bring to a simmer and let cook for 3 hours. Monitor the water closely, to make sure there is always water in the pan. Remove can from heat and let cool for 10 to 15 minutes.

Carefully open can and pour contents into pie crust. Slice bananas over the top and cool in the refrigerator. Before serving, spread with whipped topping.

Banana Oatmeal Cookies I

Ingredients

1 cup white sugar
1 cup margarine
2 eggs
1 teaspoon vanilla extract
2 cups all-purpose flour
1 teaspoon baking soda
1 teaspoon ground cloves
1 teaspoon ground cinnamon
3 ripe bananas, mashed
2 cups rolled oats
1 cup semisweet chocolate chips

Directions

Preheat oven to 375 degrees F (190 degrees C).

In a medium bowl, cream butter and sugar together until smooth. Stir in the eggs and vanilla. Sift together the flour, baking soda, cloves and cinnamon, stir into the creamed mixture. Then add the mashed bananas, rolled oats and chocolate chips, mix until well blended.

Drop dough by rounded spoonfuls onto unprepared cookie sheets. Bake for 10 to 12 minutes in the preheated oven. Remove cookies from pan to cool on wire racks.

Bananas Foster over Puff Pastry

Ingredients

1 sheet Pepperidge Farm® Puff Pastry
6 medium bananas, peeled 1/2 cup packed brown sugar 1/4 cup rum
2 tablespoons butter or margarine
1 tablespoon lemon juice
1/2 teaspoon ground cinnamon
1 cup sour cream
1 tablespoon packed brown sugar

Directions

Thaw pastry sheet at room temperature 30 minutes. Preheat oven to 425 degrees F.

Unfold pastry sheet on lightly floured surface. Trim pastry to make 9-inch circle. Place on baking sheet. Bake 10 min. or until golden. Remove from baking sheet and cool on wire rack.

Cut bananas in half lengthwise and then crosswise into slices.

Mix 1/2 cup brown sugar, rum, butter, lemon juice and cinnamon in skillet. Heat to a boil. Cook and stir until mixture thickens, about 2 min. Add bananas and toss to coat.

Mix sour cream and remaining brown sugar. Spoon banana mixture over pastry. Top with sour cream mixture. Cut into wedges.

Classic Banana Bread

Ingredients

1/4 cup butter, softened
1 cup sugar
1 cup mashed fully ripe bananas
1 cup BREAKSTONE'S Reduced
Fat Sour Cream
2 eggs
2 1/4 cups flour
1 1/2 teaspoons CALUMET
Baking Powder
1/2 teaspoon baking soda
1/2 teaspoon salt
1 cup chopped PLANTERS
Walnuts

Directions

Heat oven to 350 degrees F. Beat butter and sugar in large bowl with mixer until well blended. Add bananas, sour cream and eggs; mix well. Add combined dry ingredients; mix just until moistened. Stir in nuts.

Pour into greased and floured 9x5-inch loaf pan.

Bake 1 hour or until toothpick inserted in center comes out clean. Cool 5 minutes; remove from pan to wire rack. Cool completely before slicing to serve. Refrigerate leftovers.

Banana Chip Muffins I

Ingredients

1 3/4 cups all-purpose flour
1/2 cup white sugar
1 tablespoon baking powder
1/2 teaspoon salt
1/2 cup semisweet chocolate chips
1 egg
1/4 cup vegetable oil
1/4 cup milk
1 cup mashed bananas

Directions

Measure flour, sugar, baking powder, salt, and chocolate chips into a large bowl. Mix thoroughly, and make a well in the center.

Beat the egg in a small bowl until frothy. Mix in cooking oil, milk, and bananas. Pour mixture into the well. Stir only to moisten. Batter will be lumpy. Fill greased muffin cups 3/4 full.

Bake at 400 degrees F (205 degrees C) for 20 to 25 minutes.

Vanilla Banana French Toast

Ingredients

2 eggs
3/4 teaspoon vanilla extract
1 tablespoon ground cinnamon
2 1/4 teaspoons white sugar
2 slices bread
1 banana, sliced

Directions

Beat eggs, vanilla, cinnamon, and sugar together in a bowl. Place bread into the egg mixture to soak.

Heat a lightly oiled skillet over medium heat and brown the slices of bread on both sides. Heat a smaller lightly oiled skillet over medium-low heat and pour the remaining egg mixture into the skillet. Allow the eggs to set in the skillet for 1 to 2 minutes, then continue to cook and stir eggs until scrambled.

Place 1 slice of toast onto a plate and top with the eggs. Layer the slices of banana over the eggs, then place the second slice of toast on top to make a sandwich.

The Best Banana Pudding

Ingredients

1 (5 ounce) package instant vanilla pudding mix
2 cups cold milk
1 (14 ounce) can sweetened condensed milk
1 tablespoon vanilla extract
1 (12 ounce) container frozen whipped topping, thawed
1 (16 ounce) package vanilla wafers
14 bananas, sliced

Directions

In a large mixing bowl, beat pudding mix and milk 2 minutes. Blend in condensed milk until smooth. Stir in vanilla and fold in whipped topping. Layer wafers, bananas and pudding mixture in a glass serving bowl. Chill until serving.

Bananas Foster Ice Cream

Ingredients

1 ripe banana
1/3 cup SPLENDA® Brown Sugar Blend
1/4 cup spiced rum
1 fluid ounce banana liqueur
1 1/2 cups lowfat evaporated milk
2 cups low-fat milk
1 1/2 teaspoons almond extract
1 (3.5 ounce) package instant French vanilla pudding

Directions

Cut the banana into a few pieces and place in the bowl of a food processor along with the brown sugar blend, rum, and banana liquor. Pulse until smooth. Pour in the evaporated milk, low-fat milk, almond extract, and vanilla pudding; pulse until evenly blended. Pour into a bowl and refrigerate at least 30 minutes.

Transfer the chilled banana mixture to the cylinder of an ice cream maker; freeze according to manufacturer's directions.

Liz's Banana Bars

Ingredients

3/4 cup milk
1 teaspoon lemon juice
1/2 cup margarine, softened
1 1/2 cups white sugar
2 eggs
1/2 teaspoon salt
2 cups all-purpose flour
2 bananas, mashed

2 (3 ounce) packages cream cheese, softened
2 1/2 cups confectioners' sugar
1/3 cup margarine or butter, softened

Directions

Preheat an oven to 375 degrees F (190 degrees C). Grease a 9x13-inch baking dish.

Combine the milk and lemon juice in a small bowl; allow to sit at room temperature for 10 minutes. This will effectively 'sour' the milk.

Stir the 1/2 cup margarine, the white sugar, eggs, salt, and flour together in a bowl. Add the soured milk and mashed bananas and mix thoroughly; spread into the bottom of the prepared dish.

Bake in the preheated oven until the edges begin to brown very slightly, about 25 minutes. Allow to cool at least 10 minutes before frosting.

Prepare the frosting by beating together the cream cheese, confectioners' sugar, and 1/3 cup margarine in a bowl using an electric mixer. Spread evenly over the cooled bars before cutting into 20 even-sized pieces. Serve immediately or store in refrigerator.

Banana Fritters

Ingredients

2 ripe bananas
2 tablespoons milk
2 eggs
1 tablespoon margarine, melted
1 cup all-purpose flour
3 tablespoons white sugar
1 teaspoon baking powder
1/2 teaspoon salt
1/4 teaspoon ground cinnamon
1 pinch ground nutmeg
1 quart oil for frying
1 cup confectioners' sugar for dusting

Directions

In a large bowl, mash the bananas. Mix in milk, eggs and margarine until smooth. In a separate bowl, combine flour, sugar, baking powder, salt, cinnamon and nutmeg. Stir dry ingredients into banana mixture.

Heat oil in a deep fryer or heavy bottomed pan to 375 degrees F (190 degrees C). Drop batter by spoonfuls into hot oil, and cook, turning once, until browned, 2 to 8 minutes. Drain on paper towels and dust with confectioners' sugar.

Banana Oatmeal Cookies III

Ingredients

1 1/2 cups all-purpose flour
1 cup white sugar
1/2 teaspoon baking soda
1 teaspoon salt
1/4 teaspoon ground nutmeg 3/4
teaspoon ground cinnamon 3/4
cup shortening
1 egg, beaten
1 cup mashed ripe bananas
1 3/4 cups rolled oats
1/2 cup chopped walnuts

Directions

Preheat the oven to 400 degrees F (200 degrees C).

In a large bowl, stir together the flour, sugar, baking soda, salt, cinnamon and nutmeg. Cut in shortening until almost no lumps remain. Stir in the egg and bananas; mix well. Finally, stir in the oats and walnuts. Drop by teaspoonfuls 2 inches apart onto ungreased cookie sheets.

Bake for 12 to 15 minutes in the preheated oven, or until edges are browned. Remove from pans immediately to cool on wire racks.

Chocolate-Cherry-Banana Breakfast Smoothie

Ingredients

3 small frozen bananas (peel before you freeze)
2 cups frozen dark sweet cherries
2 cups chocolate soy milk

Directions

Place all ingredients in a blender. Blend on puree (or the highest setting) until smooth, about 30 seconds. Pour into glasses and serve.

Janet's Rich Banana Bread

Ingredients

1/2 cup butter, melted
1 cup white sugar
2 eggs
1 teaspoon vanilla extract
1 1/2 cups all-purpose flour
1 teaspoon baking soda
1/2 teaspoon salt
1/2 cup sour cream
1/2 cup chopped walnuts
2 medium bananas, sliced

Directions

Preheat oven to 350 degrees F (175 degrees C). Grease a 9x5 inch loaf pan.

In a large bowl, stir together the melted butter and sugar. Add the eggs and vanilla, mix well. Combine the flour, baking soda and salt, stir into the butter mixture until smooth. Finally, fold in the sour cream, walnuts and bananas. Spread evenly into the prepared pan.

Bake at 350 degrees F (175 degrees C) for 60 minutes, or until a toothpick inserted into the center of the loaf comes out clean. Cool loaf in the pan for 10 minutes before removing to a wire rack to cool completely.

Banana-Date Muffins

Ingredients

2 1/8 cups all-purpose flour
2 tablespoons baking powder 1/2
teaspoon ground cinnamon 1/2
teaspoon salt
1/2 cup sugar
1/2 cup reduced-calorie margarine 1
egg
3 medium ripe bananas, mashed
1 1/2 teaspoons vanilla extract
3/4 cup bran flakes cereal
12 dates, pitted and chopped

Directions

Preheat the oven to 400 degrees F (200 degrees C). Grease a muffin pan with non-stick spray or line with paper muffin liners. Sift together the flour, baking powder, cinnamon and salt; set aside.

In a medium bowl, cream together the sugar, margarine and egg with an electric mixer until light and fluffy. Mix in bananas, vanilla, cereal and dates. Blend in dry ingredients until just incorporated. Spoon into prepared muffin cups to about 2/3 full.

Bake for 20 to 25 minutes in the preheated oven, until a toothpick inserted into the center comes out clean. Cool in pan over a wire rack for at least 10 minutes before removing muffins from the pan.

Uncooked Banana Pudding

Ingredients

8 ounces sour cream
1 (8 ounce) container frozen whipped topping, thawed
1 (5 ounce) package instant vanilla pudding mix
2 cups whole milk
1 (16 ounce) package vanilla wafer cookies
4 bananas, peeled and sliced

Directions

In large bowl combine sour cream, whipped topping, pudding mix and milk. Stir well. In the bottom of a trifle bowl or other glass serving dish, put a layer of cookies, then a layer of pudding mixture, then a layer of bananas. Repeat until all ingredients are used. Refrigerate until serving.

Banana Chai Bread

Ingredients

1 3/4 cups all-purpose flour
1 tablespoon baking powder
1/2 teaspoon salt
3/4 cup white sugar
1/2 cup lowfat cream cheese
2 eggs
3/4 cup mashed bananas
1/4 cup brewed chai tea

Directions

In a medium bowl mix together flour, baking powder, and salt.

In a separate bowl mix sugar, cream cheese, and eggs until light and fluffy. Mix mashed bananas and Chai into cream cheese mixture. Add flour mixture and mix until smooth.

Pour mixture into a greased 9x5 inch loaf pan.

Bake in a preheated 350 degree F(175 degrees C) oven for 60 minutes. Cool on rack. Remove from pan after 10 minutes.

Brown Sugar Banana Bread

Ingredients

4 ripe bananas, cut into chunks
1 1/4 cups light brown sugar
1/2 cup butter, softened
1 egg
1 teaspoon cinnamon
1 teaspoon vanilla extract
1/4 cup whole milk
2 cups all-purpose flour
1/2 teaspoon baking soda
1 teaspoon baking powder
1/2 teaspoon kosher salt

Directions

Preheat oven to 350 degrees F (175 degrees C). Grease a 9x5-inch loaf pan.

Place the bananas into a large plastic zipper bag, seal the bag, and smoosh the bananas with your fingers until very well mashed. Set the bananas aside. Place the brown sugar and butter into a mixing bowl, and mix on medium speed with an electric mixer until light and fluffy, 1 to 2 minutes. Cut a corner from the plastic bag, and squeeze the mashed bananas into the bowl of brown sugar mixture. With the electric mixer on medium speed, beat in the bananas, egg, cinnamon, vanilla extract, and milk until the mixture is well combined. Switch the mixer to low speed, and gradually beat in the flour, baking soda, baking powder, and kosher salt just until the batter is smooth, about 1 minute. Spread the batter into the prepared loaf pan.

Bake in the preheated oven until the bread is set and lightly browned on top, about 40 minutes. A toothpick inserted into the center of the loaf should come out clean.

Banana Loaf

Ingredients

1/2 cup butter
1 cup white sugar
2 eggs
3 ripe bananas, mashed
2 cups all-purpose flour
1 teaspoon baking soda
1 teaspoon baking powder
1/2 teaspoon salt
1/2 cup chopped walnuts

Directions

Preheat oven to 350 degrees F (175 degrees C). Lightly grease a 9x5 inch loaf pan.

In a large bowl, cream together the butter and sugar until light and fluffy. Stir in the eggs one at a time, beating well with each addition, stir in the mashed bananas.

In a large bowl, sift together flour, baking powder, baking soda, salt. Blend the banana mixture into the flour mixture; stirring just to combine. Fold in the nuts.

Bake in preheated oven for 60 minutes, until a toothpick inserted into center of the loaf comes out clean.

Bananas in Caramel Sauce

Ingredients

1/2 cup butter
1 cup superfine sugar
1 1/4 cups heavy cream
4 bananas, peeled and halved lengthwise

Directions

In a large, heavy skillet over medium heat, melt butter. Stir in sugar and cook, stirring, until sugar is melted and light brown. Slowly stir in the cream (mixture will bubble up). Let boil 1 minute, then reduce heat to low. Place the bananas in the pan and cook until heated through, 2 minutes. Serve hot.

Aunt Betty's Banana Pudding

Ingredients

2 (3.4 ounce) packages instant vanilla pudding mix
1 cup milk
1 (14 ounce) can sweetened condensed milk
1 (8 ounce) container sour cream
1 (8 ounce) container frozen whipped topping, thawed
6 bananas, sliced
1/2 (12 ounce) package vanilla wafers

Directions

In a medium bowl, combine pudding mix and milk and stir until mix is dissolved. Refrigerate 15 minutes, until partially set.

Stir condensed milk into pudding mixture until smooth. Fold in sour cream and whipped topping. Fold in bananas.

Make a single layer of vanilla wafers in the bottom of a 9x13 inch dish. Spread pudding evenly over wafers. Crush remaining wafers and sprinkle on top. Refrigerate until serving.

Banana Fruit Mini Loaves

Ingredients

2 eggs
2/3 cup sugar
1 cup mashed bananas
1 3/4 cups all-purpose flour
3 teaspoons baking powder
1/2 teaspoon salt
1 cup mixed candied fruit
1/2 cup raisins
1/2 cup chopped walnuts

Directions

In a mixing bowl, beat eggs and sugar. Add bananas; mix well. Combine the flour, baking powder and salt; gradually add to egg mixture. Fold in fruit, raisins and walnuts. Transfer to three greased 5-3/4-in. x 3-in. x 2-in. loaf pans. Bake at 350 degrees F for 30-35 minutes or until a toothpick comes out clean. Cool for 10 minutes before removing from pans to wire racks to cool completely.

Banana Mallow Pie

Ingredients

1 3/4 cups cold milk
1 pkg. (4 serving size) JELL-O Vanilla Flavor Instant Pudding & Pie Filling
2 cups JET-PUFFED Miniature Marshmallows
1 cup thawed COOL WHIP Whipped Topping
2 medium bananas, sliced
1 (6 ounce) HONEY MAID Graham Pie Crust

Directions

Pour milk into large bowl. Add pudding mix; beat with wire whisk 2 minutes. Let stand 5 minutes. Add marshmallows and whipped topping; stir gently until well blended.

Place banana slices in crust; cover with pudding mixture.

Refrigerate at least 1 hour. Cut into 8 slices to serve. Store leftover pie in refrigerator.

Sweet Cottage Cheese and Bananas

Ingredients

1/2 cup cottage cheese
2 teaspoons honey
1 banana, sliced

Directions

In a small serving bowl, stir together the cottage cheese, honey, and banana slices. Serve or eat immediately.

Banana Cake III

Ingredients

1 cup white sugar
2 cups all-purpose flour
2 teaspoons baking soda
1/2 cup water
1 cup mashed bananas
1 pinch salt
1 cup mayonnaise
1 (8 ounce) package cream cheese
1 cup butter, softened
4 cups confectioners' sugar
2 teaspoons vanilla extract
3/4 cup chopped walnuts (optional)

Directions

Preheat oven to 350 degrees F (175 degrees C). Lightly grease two 9 inch round pans.

Combine sugar, flour, baking soda, water, mashed bananas, salt, and mayonnaise. Mix together, and pour into the cake pans.

Bake cake about 45 minutes, or until a toothpick inserted in the center comes out clean. Remove from oven, and cool on wire racks.

In a mixing bowl, blend cream cheese and butter or margarine together. Gradually add sugar and vanilla, and mix well. Stir in nuts. Fill and frost the cake.

Yuletide Banana Bread

Ingredients

1 cup whole macadamia nuts, divided
1/2 cup butter, softened
1 cup sugar
2 eggs
1 1/2 cups all-purpose flour
1 teaspoon baking soda
1/4 teaspoon salt
1 cup mashed ripe bananas
1/2 cup raisins
1/2 cup flaked coconut

Directions

In a food processor or blender, process 1/2 cup macadamia nuts until ground; set aside. Chop remaining nuts; set aside. In a mixing bowl, cream butter and sugar. Add eggs, one at a time, beating well after each addition. Combine the flour, baking soda, salt and ground nuts; stir into creamed mixture just until moistened. Fold in bananas, raisins, coconut and chopped nuts

Pour into a greased 9-in. x 5-in. x 3-in. loaf pan. Bake at 350 degrees F for 65-70 minutes or until a toothpick comes out clean. Cool for 10 minutes before removing from pan to a wire rack.

Banana Blueberry Pie

Ingredients

1 (8 ounce) package cream cheese, softened
1 cup white sugar
1 (1.3 ounce) envelope dry whipped topping mix
3 bananas, sliced
2 (9 inch) pie shells, baked
1 (21 ounce) can blueberry pie filling
1 (12 ounce) container frozen whipped topping, thawed

Directions

In a large bowl, mix together the cream cheese and sugar until light. Prepare the whipped topping mix according to package instructions, and fold into the cream cheese mixture.

Place a layer of sliced banana into the bottom of each pie shell. Spoon half of the cream cheese mixture into each pie, and spread evenly. Spoon half of the blueberry pie filling over each pie in an even layer. Cover the tops of the pies with the thawed frozen whipped topping. Chill until serving.

Really Rich Banana Bread

Ingredients

1 cup unsalted butter
1 cup dark brown sugar
6 eggs
2 cups all-purpose flour
2 teaspoons baking powder
1/4 teaspoon ground nutmeg
1 pinch ground allspice
1 pinch salt
3 ripe bananas, mashed
1 teaspoon vanilla extract

Directions

Preheat oven to 350 degrees F (175 degrees C). Grease and flour a 9x5 inch loaf pan.

In a large bowl, cream together the butter and sugar until light and fluffy. Stir in the eggs one at a time, beating well with each addition. In a separate bowl, stir together flour, baking powder, nutmeg, allspice and salt. Blend the flour mixture into the butter and egg mixture a bit at a time, beating well after each addition.. Stir in the banana and vanilla; mixing just enough to evenly combine. Pour batter into prepared pan.

Bake in preheated oven for 90 minutes, until a toothpick inserted into center of the loaf comes out clean. Cool the cake in the pan for 10 minutes and then turn out onto a wire rack to cool completely.

Fluffy Banana Cake

Ingredients

2 bananas, broken into chunks
2 cups sifted all-purpose flour
1/2 teaspoon baking powder
3/4 teaspoon baking soda
1/2 teaspoon salt
1/2 cup shortening
1 1/2 cups white sugar
2 eggs
1 teaspoon vanilla extract
1/4 cup buttermilk
4 cups whipped heavy cream

Directions

Preheat oven to 350 degrees F (175 degrees C). Grease and flour two 9 inch layer cake pans. Sift together flour, baking powder, soda, and salt; set aside.

In a large bowl, combine the shortening, sugar, eggs, and vanilla. Beat well. Blend in the buttermilk. Add sifted flour mixture alternately with mashed banana to the egg mixture while beating. Pour batter into prepared pans.

Bake cake for 30 to 35 minutes. Remove from pans, and cool on wire racks. Fill and frost the cake with whipped cream.

CPSIA information can be obtained
at www.ICGtesting.com
Printed in the USA
BVHW011558070621
608939BV00013B/2380